The Know-how
of Breast-feeding

The Know-how of Breast-feeding

Sylvia Close
S.A.N.C. Med. and Surg. (Hons.)
S.A.N.C. Midwifery (Hons.)
Athlone Mothercraft Certificate
in Infant Dietetics

 Bristol
John Wright & Sons Ltd.
1972. Reprinted 1979

COPYRIGHT NOTICE

© SYLVIA CLOSE

BY THE SAME AUTHOR

The Know-how of Infant Feeding
The Know-how of Infant Care
The Know-how of Pregnancy and Labour
(Bristol: John Wright & Sons Ltd.)

First published 1972
Reprinted 1976
Reprinted 1979

ISBN 0 7236 0324 3

PRINTED IN GREAT BRITAIN BY HENRY LING LTD., A SUBSIDIARY OF JOHN WRIGHT AND SONS LTD., AT THE DORSET PRESS, DORCHESTER

INTRODUCTION

Most intelligent women want to breast-feed their babies, and if all goes well breast-feeding can be easy and enjoyable. Unfortunately, problems and difficulties do crop up in the early days and weeks of the baby's life, making the new mother anxious and concerned.

What the mother then needs is an understanding of what is causing the problems and difficulties, together with guidance on how to deal with them. If she does not get this sort of help, and the particular problem is not corrected quickly, then her confidence will be undermined and she will become more and more anxious, upset, and depressed.

A chain reaction will follow—her emotional state will lead to fatigue, exhaustion, less breast-milk, a hungry, crying baby, and a mother who feels guilty and inadequate.

For most people, unfortunately, the only solution to this state of affairs is bottle-feeding, which is such a pity and is so unnecessary.

The aims of this little book are:—

1. To help women to breast-feed happily.
2. To encourage those who have doubts, in favour of breast-feeding.
3. To give women an understanding of the subject.
4. To help them correct the problems which might otherwise lead to unnecessarily abandoning breast-feeding in favour of bottle-feeding.

Is not bottle-feeding as good as breast-feeding?
Until recently it was thought that the advantages of breast-feeding applied only to the early phases (weeks and months) of an infant's life—when he was small and helpless, and needed his mother for nourishment, for physical and emotional security, and for protection against diseases. And as a ' reward ' the mother's internal organs benefited and returned to the normal state more quickly. But now there is increasing scientific evidence to suggest that the advantages of breast-feeding are carried into adulthood and are maintained throughout life. Thus, if you breast-feed you are likely to be laying a long-lasting solid foundation for good health in your child.

When you bottle-feed, no matter which preparation you use, you are in fact giving your baby cow's milk, either in the form of dried powder or as a concentrated liquid.

All the baby foods, correctly modified, are good substitutes, but they do not equal the biochemical perfection of breast-milk for the human baby.

Each mammal mother secretes the milk best suited to her own young, so that cow's milk is the best food for the calf, and human breast-milk is the best possible food for the human baby.

If you choose to bottle-feed you should be aware that you choose to give your baby second best. Whereas, if you breast-feed, the advantages are many. They are real and they are lasting, both for you and your baby.

4

ADVANTAGES IN INFANCY

1. The composition of breast-milk is absolutely perfect for the baby, particularly with regard to the calcium and phosphate balance and the vitamin E content.
2. Breast-milk is always at the right temperature—not too hot and not too cold.
3. Breast-milk costs nothing and so saves the family money—not only the cost of baby foods but also the cost of bottles, teats, sterilizers, bottle-warmers, etc.
4. Breast-milk is always available. It does not require any preparation, and this saves the mother time.
5. Breast-fed babies are less prone to gastro-intestinal (tummy) infections, respiratory (chest) infections, and other infections in the first year of life, as well as later.
6. Breast-feeding protects the baby against constipation. Breast-fed babies may have infrequent stools, but they are never constipated.
7. There are no irritating substances in the urine or stools of the breast-fed baby to cause nappy rash.
8. From the close contact with his mother when feeding the baby enjoys a warm, safe, secure, protected, emotional environment, and this contributes to his mental health.
9. Breast-milk aids the recovery of sick babies, because it is easier to digest than formula feeds.
10. Premature babies do better if they are fed on expressed breast-milk.

For reasons (9) and (10) some hospitals have breast-milk banks. In Helsinki, Finland, for example, breast-milk is bought from willing donors. Every day it is collected from over a wide area and brought to a children's hospital. There it is analysed, sterilized, frozen, and stored, and when needed it is used for special little patients.

11. Some authorities believe that breast-feeding protects

the baby against a tragic phenomenon known as 'sudden cot death'. Although the exact cause of this is not known it is thought to be due to either an acute virus infection, an allergy to cow's milk, or a low level of vitamin E.

12. For those who are concerned about general radiation dangers, the strontium level in breast-milk is about one-sixth of that in cow's milk.

13. Breast-feeding aids the more rapid return to normal of the mother's internal organs after pregnancy and labour.

IT IS ALSO THOUGHT THAT

1. The higher resistance of the breast-fed baby to infections is maintained throughout childhood, and possibly even throughout life.

2. Teeth tend to be stronger in the child who has been breast-fed. Studies have suggested that early weaning is associated with increased caries in pre-school children.

3. There is less likelihood of suffering from circulatory and coronary heart disease. Studies have shown that the changes in the blood-vessels begin in infancy and are associated with early bottle-feeding.

4. It is even possible that there is less risk of kidney complaints, as bottle-feeding throws a greater strain on the infant's kidneys.

5. There is less risk of obesity, as bottle-fed babies are more likely to be overweight and this may persist throughout life.

6. The mother who has breast-fed is less likely to get cancer of the breast in later life. Some authorities believe that women who have suppressed lactation, or have never lactated, are more prone to breast cancer.

Should I breast-feed even if I'm not very keen to do so?
Yes, your baby would certainly benefit from it, especially if your baby is a boy.

The female hormones protect women against coronary heart disease until after the menopause. Men, however, are not similarly protected, and as the condition is now thought to be linked with early bottle-feeding there is certainly a definite good reason to breast-feed. Even if you start breast-feeding as a duty to your baby, you may find in time that you actually enjoy the experience.

Perhaps the following quotation from a letter may encourage you:—

'. . . It seems hard to believe that it's five months since C. was born, and almost that long since I last saw you. Somehow the time has gone so quickly and so happily!

' I don't seem to have any problems or any worries: I never honestly expected it all to be so easy and such fun (and I hope I won't have to go back on these words!). But I can't tell you how grateful I am for all the advice and encouragement you gave on breast-feeding. I really wasn't at all interested at trying it when I was first pregnant—and your talks were just what I needed. I'm so glad I have. C. of course is so healthy and contented—and I'm so thrilled with it.

' There's no need I know, to try and tell you how immensely satisfying and labour-saving I've found it. But it's hard to fully understand all that it offers until you've actually done it yourself. (Like giving birth to C.—I feel as thrilled and as proud as if I was the first person to discover the experience!!) '

This baby was breast-fed for 9 months.

How can I prepare for breast-feeding before the baby is born?
Any woman with normal breasts and nipples is capable of breast-feeding her baby. A baby is able to feed from any nipple which, on stimulation, will protrude beyond the breast surface.

During pregnancy your breasts are automatically prepared without your active help as follows:—
1. The pregnancy hormones cause the glandular tissue in

7

the breasts to grow, develop, and secrete colostrum.

2. The blood-supply is increased in preparation for making breast-milk.

3. The nipples also enlarge and tend to protrude more.

ALL YOU HAVE TO DO IS

1. Support the increased weight of the breasts and prevent sagging by wearing a good supporting bra *day and night* from the onset of the pregnancy. Make sure that there is no pressure on the nipples.

2. Keep the breasts and nipples clean: nothing more need be done than your normal bath routine.

3. If the skin tends to be dry, then avoid soap and apply lanoline or massé cream as often as you need.

4. If your nipples are flat then draw them out by rolling them between your fingers. Use a little lanolin, Nivea cream, massé cream, or oil to do this.

5. If you have inverted nipples try the following three ways of correcting the condition:—

   a. Manual manipulation, as described above.

   b. Ask your doctor to prescribe special shells to wear inside your bra. (They are known as either Woolwich or Waller's Shells.)

   c. Your husband can also help to draw them out when you make love.

Note: There is no need to spend money on a special ' feeding ' chair. You can make yourself comfortable and breast-feed successfully and happily virtually anywhere —while sitting on a chair, couch, bed, etc.

Does one have to have perfect nipples to be able to breast-feed?

Not necessarily. It is, indeed, quite remarkable how a

8

new baby will adapt himself to any slight imperfections of his mother's nipples and will feed quite successfully if only he is given the chance to do so.

What is, however, important in such cases, which include small nipples, extra-large nipples, and even flat nipples, is to get the baby to the breast as soon after delivery as possible. By touching his upper lip and then his lower lip again and again with your nipple, aim to get his mouth open wide enough to enclose the whole nipple. With patient perseverance and frequent short sessions at the breast every day before the breasts become hard and engorged, you will both succeed.

The following quote from a letter should encourage any mother in a similar situation:—

'. . . Incidentally—they told me at the hospital that it was technically impossible for me to breast-feed my baby (because of the shape of my nipples) and tried to persuade me (without success) to have the hormones to dry up the milk. When I left the hospital a combination of worry and lack of stimulation had more or less dried up the milk anyway and the baby was getting 3 oz. of Cow & Gate milk each feed (at 7 days old). Not deterred, once at home we worked at getting him to suck properly and on working up the milk-supply, and the milk came in so quickly that we were able to dispense with bottles after only a fortnight.
' While I know that the nipples are not ideal, I feel that most of the trouble was due to the baby's being cot-nursed for 24 hours and in that time being given large quantities of cow's milk while not being allowed to suck at the breast. Due to his large birth-weight (8 lb. 14 oz.) he was being given $1\frac{1}{2}$ oz. per feed in his first day! '

This baby was successfully breast-fed for $8\frac{1}{2}$ months, in spite of the difficult beginning.

Is it necessary to express from my breasts during pregnancy?
It is not necessary to express the colostrum from your breasts during pregnancy for the following reasons:—
1. Colostrum is a precious substance, and the baby should get it all in the first few days of his life.

2. The reason why expressing is sometimes advised is to prevent engorgement of the breasts 3–5 days after delivery. But this condition can be treated very simply, safely, and effectively with cold compresses (*see* p. 31). Relief is obtained immediately and, if repeated according to need, then within 24 hours the engorgement will have disappeared.
3. Expressing is a skill which takes time to acquire, and one has to have a knowledge of the anatomy of the breast to prevent bruising of the glandular tissue.
4. The emotional strain associated with learning to express and the anxiety felt if nothing, or only very little, comes out may be enough to make a woman doubtful about her ability to breast-feed later on after her baby is born. This doubt may actually inhibit the normal process of lactation.

Note: Nor is it necessary to express after the baby is born. Only mothers of premature or sick babies, who cannot feed directly from the breast, should express so that their babies can benefit from the expressed breast-milk.

To express you have to empty the ampullae (sacs or reservoirs behind the nipple). They are situated in a circle where the lighter and darker skin meet.

With your thumb and middle finger on opposite sides of the circle squeeze gently and rhythmically. It will take a little while before a drop appears at the end of the nipple, and shortly after that the milk will begin to spurt.

Continue with the rhythmic squeezing, gradually increasing the pressure, until no more milk comes out. Now move your fingers around a little, so that you press on and empty other sacs. Keep moving your fingers around to new parts of the circle and repeat the rhythmic squeezing. In this way you will empty all the little reservoirs behind the nipple.

How can I be sure that I'll be able to produce enough milk?
The production of milk happens automatically after the baby is born, because of the alteration in the balance of your hormones. Milk production is perpetuated by the baby sucking. As long as the baby sucks at the breast there will be milk.

The amount of milk is determined by the frequency of feeds and the strength of the sucking. In other words, as the baby gets older he sucks more powerfully and so causes more milk to be created. A relaxed state in the mother allows the whole process to work efficiently.

So all you have to do is to feed your baby at least five times per day, making sure that he sucks properly, and relax and be confident.

Even if you have twins it is still possible to breast-feed them completely. Unfortunately, women are not often encouraged to do so, as the following quote from a letter shows:—

'I had four sisters come to see me in hospital the day I went home, plus the consultant, because they wanted to see the freak who wanted to breast-feed her twin babies.'

However, because of the mother's persistence and good sense these babies were breast-fed for 10 months.

How is the inside of the breast constructed?
Each breast is composed of about 20 branch-like structures called lobes, radiating outwards from the nipple, and separated by varying amounts of fat—hence the difference in size as between one woman and another.

These lobes are subdivided into many smaller lobules

which terminate in milk-secreting glands called alveoli or acini. The alveoli have a rich blood-supply from which the breast-milk is created. An efficient muscle structure surrounding the alveoli squeezes the breast-milk into tiny ducts leading from them.

These tiny ducts join up to form larger ducts—one for each lobule—and the larger ducts join up to one main duct for each lobe. The lobe ducts in turn lead to the nipple, but before reaching the nipple they expand to form little reservoirs or sacs known as ampullae, then they narrow again and lead into the nipple. There are muscle-fibres in the nipples which act as a sphincter, and this prevents the leaking of the milk.

The size of the breast depends on the amount of fat between the lobes and as fat does not in any way contribute to the production of milk the size of the breasts is immaterial as far as successful breast-feeding is concerned. In fact, small breasts very often work more efficiently than very heavy pendulous breasts with too much fat. It is the glandular tissue which produces the milk, and this is fairly constant for all women.

How is breast-milk produced?

After the baby is born there is a change in the hormone balance of the mother and an increase in the blood-supply to the breasts. Two hormones from the pituitary gland now influence the breasts:—

1. Prolactin is responsible for changing blood into breast-milk.
2. Oxytocin is responsible for squeezing the milk into sacs or reservoirs behind the nipple. Here the milk is stored until the baby feeds.

When the baby sucks he empties the sacs and stimulates

12

the release of oxytocin, which in turn liberates prolactin, and the whole process is repeated.

The production of milk is a continuous process which depends on, and is maintained by, the baby's sucking. The more the baby sucks the more milk will be created, and in this way the milk-supply is perpetuated according to his needs.

If two babies suck there will be more milk created than if only one baby is fed. Also, after a while milk is produced more efficiently in less time. This is why as the baby grows older he gets more milk in less time, and why there will always be milk as long as the baby continues to suck.

The more relaxed and confident you are the more efficiently will it all work. And, because the breast-milk is created from your blood the quality will always be perfect for your baby—he was also nourished by your blood before he was born.

How does the baby know what to do?

The newborn baby reacts instinctively, and it may well be that Nature meant his introduction to feeding to proceed along the following lines.

Women giving birth have sometimes been observed to stretch out their arms instinctively and to lean forward as if to grasp and support the emerging baby. If the mother were allowed to do this the baby would automatically follow the natural curve of the birth canal and land on her abdomen. The baby is born with certain automatic inborn reflexes. Apart from the *breathing reflex* which keeps him alive, the *grasping reflex* would enable him to cling to his mother. Guided by his mother the *walking reflex* would propel him forward. The *rooting reflex* would help him find the nipple, and the *sucking reflex* would enable him to get colostrum and in turn initiate the whole process of lactation.

How does the baby actually get the milk from the breast?
The baby is born with sucking pads inside his cheeks and a sucking reflex. When he grasps the nipple (between his tongue and upper palate) a vacuum is created in his mouth. The pressure in the breast is then greater than the vacuum in his mouth and this causes the milk, which is stored in the ampullae (little sacs, or reservoirs, behind the nipple), to flow into his mouth. The swallowing reflex then comes into play and his mouth is emptied. And as he sucks more milk flows into his mouth.

Also, when the baby sucks, a hormone (oxytocin) is released from the mother's pituitary gland. This hormone contracts the glandular tissue of the mother's breasts, squeezing the milk into and along the ducts which lead to the nipples.

The mother feels this activity as a drawing, draining sensation inside her breasts. This is known as the ' draught ' or ' let-down ' reflex. Doubt, anxiety, and all negative emotions can inhibit the let-down reflex, whereas an understanding of the whole process and a relaxed and confident frame of mind will aid the natural function of milk production.

How does colostrum differ from breast-milk?
Colostrum can be regarded as the bridge between the blood which nourished the baby inside the uterus before he was born, and the breast-milk which is produced a few days after his birth.

Whereas colostrum is yellowish in colour, breast-milk looks bluish-white. Colostrum contains more protein but less sugar and fat than breast-milk. There are more anti-bodies in colostrum than in breast-milk to protect the newborn baby from infections. Some authorities also believe that colostrum helps to mature the lining of the baby's bowel, making it impervious to harmful germs. And this is considered one of the reasons why breast-fed babies rarely get gastro-enteritis and are rarely involved in the epidemics which sometimes occur among newborn babies in hospitals.

Colostrum contains an aperient factor which clears the baby's bowel of meconium. Meconium is the name given to the contents of the bowel in the unborn and newly born baby. It is dark greenish-black in colour and is tacky in consistency. The first stool that a baby passes is sterile because it was created before he was born while in the sterile environment of the uterus. It is the one and only sterile stool that any individual ever has.

Breast-milk also has an aperient factor, and this is why breast-fed babies are never constipated. They may have infrequent stools (as infrequently as every 5–6 days, even) but the stools are never formed, hard, or brittle.

Will my breasts become very large while I am breast-feeding?
At puberty the breasts develop. During pregnancy they enlarge and mature in preparation for lactation.

A few days after the baby is born the breasts become engorged and increase in size. This is a temporary state and with proper care (*see* p. 31) they will settle down within a day or so to almost the pregnancy size. They remain this size throughout the breast-feeding period. After weaning they return to approximately the pre-pregnancy size.

It is advisable to keep your breasts well supported by wearing a bra not only during the day but also at night until your baby is completely weaned.

Does it hurt the mother when the baby sucks at the breast?

Not only does it *not* hurt the mother when the baby sucks but most women actually experience sexual pleasure when the baby is feeding. The possible explanation for this is that oxytocin, the hormone responsible for the ' let-down ' reflex, is thought to be also associated with the female orgasm.

What can make feeding painful is sore or cracked nipples, so try to prevent this happening—it is easier to prevent the condition than it is to cure it. Also, if the baby grasps only the tip of the nipple then it will hurt, and drawing the rest of the nipple into his mouth will hurt and predispose to cracks in the skin of the nipple. So make sure that he grasps the whole nipple correctly right from the beginning.

Something that has put many women off breast-feeding is being told that the baby has to get the whole areola (the darker skin surrounding the nipple) into his mouth ' because it is necessary for his gums to press on the sacs or reservoirs to empty them '.

This is not only unnecessary, and at times physically impossible, but the theory is quite fallacious. If the gums have to press on the sacs then it would hurt the mother, and it would be impossible to breast-feed once the teeth appear. And yet we know that in some cultures children are breast-fed for several years, when they have many if not all their baby teeth.

16

TO PREVENT SORE NIPPLES

1. Increase the time of sucking on each breast gradually every day as follows:—

1st	2nd	3rd	4th	5th	6th	7th	8th and following days
2	3	4–5	6–7	7–8	8–9	9–10	10
min.	min.	min.	min.	min.	min.	min.	min.

on each breast at every feed

2. Avoid pulling the nipple out of the baby's mouth while he is sucking. Rather, wait for the baby to pause and rest and then push it firmly to the corner of his mouth and it will slip out easily.
3. After feeds, dry the nipples carefully by dabbing them with a clean lawn handkerchief. Wet sodden nipples are much more liable to become tender and sore.
4. Make sure that when the baby grasps the nipple his mouth closes over the whole nipple and not just part of it.
5. Do not swab the nipples before or after feeds. Your daily bath or shower is quite adequate for cleaning purposes.
6. Use soap sparingly on the nipples because it tends to dissolve the protective oils in the skin, predisposing them to tenderness and cracking.
7. Do not brush the nipples or use spirits with the mistaken idea that it will toughen them. They are much more likely to be hurt by this treatment.
8. As a general rule do not allow the baby to feed for longer than 10 minutes on each breast (this includes pauses and rests).
9. Massé cream or other soothing preparations such as lanolin can be applied to the nipples after feeds as a preventive measure.

17

TO HEAL SORE NIPPLES

Treatment is a matter of trial and error as to what will heal your skin quickly. The following suggestions are worth trying:—

1. Expose your nipples to the air or sunlight for short spells 2–3 times per day.
2. Apply massé cream, cod-liver oil, or vitamin E oil to the nipples after feeds.
3. Some women find Friar's Balsam very helpful, either applied directly on to the sore part, or a few drops mixed with some soothing ointment, e.g., lanolin or massé cream.
4. Ask your doctor to prescribe an ointment.
5. If it hurts too much when the baby feeds then use a rubber nipple-shield for a while. As a rule it is only the first few seconds which are uncomfortable. For the rest of the feed there is no discomfort or pain.

But isn't breast-feeding messy?

By this you probably imagine that the lactating woman is constantly leaking milk and messing her clothes. This need never happen if you understand what is involved and what to do.

1. There are little muscles in the nipples which act as sphincters and close the openings in the nipple. If these muscles are a little lax then milk may ooze out from the sacs or reservoirs behind the nipples. To control this all you have to do is to splash cold water on to the base of the nipple and the nipple itself several times a day. This will help to tone up the muscle structure involved and prevent further leaking.
2. While the baby is sucking at one breast, milk may flow from the other breast. If this happens, cover the

18

nipple with a clean nappy and press the heel of your hand on to the nipple. This will prevent further leaking.

3. The let-down reflex (which results in milk flowing out of the glandular tissue into the ducts leading to the nipple) may be set off by any stimulus directly or indirectly associated with the baby. For this reason, when you are going out, it is wise to cover the breasts with clean handkerchiefs and squares of polythene before putting on your bra. It may happen that if you are away from your baby and see that is nearly feeding time, or you hear a baby cry, or someone enquires about your baby—any of these may be enough to stimulate the let-down reflex. But the leak will not show if you have prepared yourself.

Can breast-milk suddenly disappear?

Once lactation has been established and your breasts are being stimulated by the baby's sucking you will continue to create milk and it is physically impossible for the milk to disappear suddenly.

Shock and emotional upsets may disrupt the normal functioning, reduce the amount of milk, and inhibit the let-down reflex. But this is a temporary phase and you can work up the milk-supply again quite easily. To re-assure you further just bear in mind that in order to inhibit or stop lactation, women not only avoid active stimulation by not breast-feeding but they are also given hormones or other medication. Sometimes the treatment has to be repeated to dry up the milk completely.

Also, women who have weaned naturally (without the aid of drugs) find that many months later—even 6–7 months later—they still have some milk left in their breasts.

So, when somebody tells you that she woke up one morning and there wasn't a drop of milk left in her breasts, she is mistaken. She came to this erroneous conclusion either because she tried to express and did not do it quite correctly, or because her breasts had settled down and were no longer hard and engorged and therefore she mistakenly assumed that they were empty.

Is breast-feeding tiring?

There is no need to anticipate or expect to feel tired when you breast-feed, as very little physical effort is involved. In fact, if you were bottle-feeding you would have to spend much more time and effort in preparing feeds and cleaning bottles.

When women who breast-feed complain of being tired and exhausted it is due almost entirely to emotional causes:—

1. Doubt as to whether the baby is getting enough milk.
2. Lack of confidence in handling the baby.
3. Indecision as to what is best for the baby.
4. General anxieties and worries.
5. Inability to understand and to know how to comfort the baby.
6. Distress when the baby cries.

These emotions also react through the autonomic nervous system and inhibit the normal process of lactation. This, in turn, results in less breast-milk and therefore a hungry crying baby and a more distressed and tired mother.

Thus it is not necessarily lots of extra physical rest which a new mother needs. What is much more important is that she should be emotionally secure and confident about her natural ability to feed her baby.

20

Let us analyse what actual effort is involved and how you can minimize it:—

1. You can make sure that each feeding session will last no more than 30 minutes. Of this, only 20 minutes will be devoted to actual breast-feeding, i.e., 10 minutes on each breast. This 10 minutes includes any pauses and rests. In fact, the baby gets most of what he needs in the first 4–5 minutes on each breast. The remaining 10 minutes will be spent changing the nappy and putting the baby down to sleep. This you will have to do anyway, whether you breast-feed or bottle-feed.

2. As you will be giving your baby 5–6 feeds in 24 hours, feeding time will occupy in total only $2\frac{1}{2}$–3 hours of your day.

3. If you consciously relax while feeding your baby, then each feed becomes a period of rest rather than a tiring chore.

Now that you know what to aim for, try to put it into practice and then, instead of getting tired, you will enjoy feeding your baby.

Is it necessary to stop breast-feeding if I become emotionally upset?

No, certainly not. Most women are bound to have some emotional upsets during the 9 months of breast-feeding, but as these states are of short duration the effect will be temporary.

What, however, is much more damaging is doubt and anxiety which persists over days, or even weeks.

WHAT TO DO IF YOU HAVE BEEN UPSET

1. Before each feed sit down and relax for a while. It will help if you do gentle, slow breathing at the

same time, taking a little longer over breathing out.

2. Reassure the baby with your voice by talking to him softly, slowly, and soothingly. Tell him that you are sorry that he is not getting enough today but you have been upset, and tomorrow he will get more.

3. If necessary give him a few extra sessions at the breast, even if only for 5 minutes on each side.

4. Be confident that he will not starve, even if he is going a little short for a day.

5. Above all do not panic and do not start bottle-feeding.

6. Do all your housework and chores in a relaxed way, slowly and happily, and without urgency and strain. This will help you to recover more quickly because if if you are relaxed you cannot at the same time be emotionally upset. The two states are diametrically opposed to each other.

7. If necessary work up your milk-supply (*see* p. 52).

8. If you have been anxious for some time you will need to have your confidence restored, and for this you will need reassurance from some other sympathetic person, such as your antenatal teacher or a friend who has breast-fed successfully.

Should I avoid certain foods while I am breast-feeding?
No! Continue with your normal diet which should consist of small helpings of a large variety of foods to give you all that you nutritionally require. It is unlikely that any food in small or normal quantities which agrees with you will affect the baby adversely.

If the baby develops a spotty skin it may be due to a high fat content in your breast-milk. To correct this cut down on the following items in your diet: chocolates, sweets, sugars, jams, and other starchy foods, as well as cocoa and chocolate drinks.

Women have often been told to avoid certain foods, e.g., oranges, grapes, strawberries, etc., but this is quite unnecessary. Bear in mind that women who live in fruit-growing countries and eat these fruits in much larger quantities are still able to breast-feed, and their babies do no suffer in any way.

However, if you are convinced that a specific food does upset the baby then leave it out of your diet for a while and reintroduce it (a very small amount) a few weeks later, gradually working up the amount to a normal portion. Or leave it out altogether and find a substitute for it.

Is it true that some women can and some women cannot breast-feed?

All women are potentially capable of breast-feeding. The physiological changes predisposing to lactation occur in all women after the termination of a pregnancy—not only after the birth of a baby but also after a miscarriage or an abortion. After a difficult labour or a Caesarean delivery the process takes a little longer, and breast-milk may not be available for the first 5–6 days. Whether the woman will breast-feed or not depends on two main factors:—

1. *Her emotional state and her attitude to breast-feeding*

She is more likely to succeed if she is happy, relaxed, and confident, and has her husband's support. Encouragement from close relatives and friends also helps. She is less likely to succeed if she is ' neurotic ' about breast-feeding: either repelled or reluctant on the one hand, or frantically urgent and determined to succeed on the other.

23

2. *Whether the physiological state is handled correctly*

If all is well and the baby feeds properly and there are no problems she is more likely to continue breast-feeding. But bottle-feeding will seem to her a happier alternative if:—

a. The first feeds are mismanaged, and both mother and baby are reduced to tears.

b. Engorged breasts are massaged, expressed, or in any other way hurt.

c. The nipples are allowed to become tender, sore, or cracked, and the mother suffers pain at every feed.

d. Unnecessary bottle-feeds are given to the new-born baby and he is too sleepy to suck at feeding times. Then each feed becomes a struggle and the mother becomes discouraged, frustrated, and upset because the baby does not feed properly.

e. The mother is told that she does not have enough breast-milk for her baby—' he is a big baby and he needs more '. There is still the tendency to assess the baby's requirements according to his weight rather than his age. This shatters the woman's confidence, makes her feel guilty and inadequate, and actually inhibits the normal process of lactation.

Assuming that a baby gets 5 feeds in 24 hours, his approximate requirements per feed are:—

1st day	2nd day	3rd day	4th day	5th day	6th day	7th day	8th day
Colustrum	Colostrum	¼ oz.	½ oz.	¾ oz.	1 oz.	1¼ oz.	1½ oz.

9th day	10th day	11th day	12th day	13th day	14th day	3rd week	4th week
1¾ oz.	2 oz.	2¼ oz.	2½ oz.	2¾ oz.	3 oz.	3½ oz.	4 oz.

1st month	2nd month	3rd month	4th month	5th month	6th, month	7th, 8th, 9th
4½ oz.	5 oz.	5½ oz.	6 oz.	6½ oz.	7 oz.	

So, you see, if a woman does not breast-feed it is not necessarily because she is incapable of breast-feeding but because her introduction to breast-feeding was mismanaged. Any woman who succeeds in breast-feeding today in spite of such obstacles is quite remarkable and is to be congratulated.

Note: Only a small percentage of women—those who have anatomical abnormalities such as inverted nipples or abnormally large and pendulous breasts—will have difficulty with breast-feeding. The first group can produce an adequate milk-supply but the baby is incapable of getting it. The second group do lactate but not efficiently, and the baby would possibly require complementary bottle-feeding as well.

Then there are women who although they are physically capable of breast-feeding are advised against it for medical reasons because they suffer from some debilitating disease.

I failed to breast-feed my first baby. Am I likely to succeed with another baby?
As long as you have normal breasts and nipples, and the babies are capable of sucking, you can breast-feed all your subsequent babies.

Your increased knowledge and understanding will give you confidence in managing the feeds and so help you to succeed.

QUOTE FROM A LETTER
' My reason for failing to breast-feed my first child, a boy, was being unable to get him to suck properly because of my lack of knowledge of the physical facts about sucking and the way to hold the baby properly.
' I was also unfortunate in that I lacked confidence as well as knowledge and the midwives and doctor, although very patient,

were rather on the side of bottle-feeding, and of course I felt that they must know best. So faced with a hungry baby I gave in and bottle-fed him. I believe my failure was mainly due to lack of instruction before the birth (all feeding instruction was about bottle-feeding) and lack of confidence in myself. At the clinic breast-feeding was regarded as a difficult, inconvenient, unconventional method by all the other mothers and was virtually ignored by those responsible for instruction. Most books I read while pregnant had a similar view-point.

' The second time I became pregnant I was given quite a different approach to pregnancy, childbirth, and feeding, and as a result I have breast-fed my second child, a girl, so far for 8 months.

' ... On many occasions I felt a great regret for not having breast-fed my first child. . . .

' . . . I should like to mention that I have had two holidays while breast-feeding and have found it quick, clean, convenient, and unobtrusive—bottle-feeding being the opposite.'

Since breast-milk appears only on the third day after birth, how does the baby survive until then?

The normal baby is born with a ' nutritional hump ', i.e., he has a store of glycogen in his liver and his muscles and so needs very little extra nourishment for the first few days. The bigger the baby the larger is his ' nutritional hump '.

Also, when put to the breast in the first few days the baby gets a substance called colostrum, which has a high protein content and is easy for the newborn baby to digest. That is why a small amount of it, even only 1–2 teaspoons per feed, is enough for the baby until the breast-milk becomes available.

Note: Sick babies, or the immature baby whose mother has diabetes (although heavy at birth), require special care and special feeding.

How can I manage the first feed if no one helps me?

It is advisable to get the baby to suck at the breast as soon after he is born as possible in order to exercise and strengthen the sucking reflex.

26

In fact there is no reason why after a normal labour you should not put him to the breast while you are still on the delivery table and waiting for the placenta to be expelled.

It is important to be in a relaxed and happy frame of mind and to avoid distress, frustration, and fatigue. If you are prevented from doing so while on the delivery table, do not insist and get upset but wait until the baby is brought to you several hours later when you are comfortably settled in bed in your own room.

HOW TO PROCEED

1. Sit bolt upright and make yourself comfortable in the sitting position, but do not lean back on the pillows because you will not be able to control the whole proceeding.
2. Undo your bra.
3. Loosen the baby's wrapping blanket. This will help to wake him if he is asleep.
4. Supporting the baby's head and shoulders with one hand, lift him up and sit him on your lap. Now lean him back and let his head rest in the bend of your elbow.
5. Touch the corner of his mouth which is nearer to you either with your nipple or your finger and he will turn his head in that direction, which is towards your body. This is called the 'rooting reflex'.
6. Support the breast with your free hand and get him to open his mouth by touching his upper lip and then his lower lip with the nipple. It may be necessary to repeat this several times before he opens his mouth.
7. As soon as his mouth is open move his head nearer towards you so that his open mouth closes over the

nipple. It requires a little practice to get the timing right, but you have all the time in the world, so do not get upset if his mouth closes before he has grasped the nipple. Repeat steps (6) and (7) patiently until he gets the nipple.

8. He will automatically start sucking. Allow him to do so for 2 minutes only.

9. While he is sucking, lean forward and watch him, making sure that you are quite relaxed. Check that your shoulders are not hunched, that your elbow is well supported, and that your wrists and hands are not stiff. (Sitting in a stiff, tense way will tire you.)

10. If his nose is pressed against the breast and this interferes with his breathing, gently lower the elbow which is supporting his head. He will then have a clear airway and so be able to suck properly. There is no need to press into the breast tissue with a finger or you may compress the ducts inside the breast.

11. After letting him suck for 2 minutes wait until he pauses and then push the nipple firmly with your finger to the corner of his mouth and it will slip out easily. Never pull the nipple out of his mouth as this may cause sore or cracked nipples.

12. Dab the nipple dry with a clean lawn handkerchief which you keep in your bra for this purpose.

13. Repeat all this on the other side.

Note: Always wait for a pause before removing the nipple from his mouth. Never, never pull the nipple out while he is still sucking.

QUOTE FROM A REPORT

'. . . Getting the baby to the breast is another point; there were only two people on the ward I found helpful, a nursery nurse and a sister. The rest when they came to see how one was getting on, held the baby's head, my nipple, and pushed him and it together!! However, when one is feeding well, they are very proud of the fact that you are breast-feeding and that it is all thanks to them!

' At one feeding time a sister tutor and three nurses came round the ward to see how everyone was getting on. She said I looked very relaxed and was managing very well—had I read anything about breast-feeding? I told her all about you and the Trust and your books. She was most impressed. I also told her that everyone working on the ward had a different view on feeding, and that if one hadn't read something about it, you would be overcome with confusion.

' I can honestly say that if I didn't know you and if I hadn't read and re-read you book (*The Know-how of Infant Feeding*) I, too, would have a bottle-fed baby.'

I am very keen to breast-feed my baby but I believe sometimes the hospital staff persuade mothers to bottle-feed. What shall I do if it happens to me?

In any conflict with the professional staff in hospital you are obviously at a great disadvantage. But it is your baby and you have the right to feed him the way you wish, e.g., if you were a vegetarian then no one could persuade you to give your child meat. So, assuming that all is well and that you and your baby are both perfectly healthy then similarly you can insist on breast-feeding.

The more you know about the subject of breast-feeding the better prepared you are to understand and cope with any difficulties that may crop up, and no matter what happens in hospital (even if the baby is bottle-fed) you can correct it when you come home (*see* p. 34). You can refuse to take drugs to dry up your breast-milk and can reasonably point out that if you do not have any breast-milk you do not need drugs to dry up what you have not got. On the other hand, if you do have some breast-milk then you want your baby to have it, no matter how little there is. If necessary you will give him a complementary feed as well. When you come home you can work up the milk-supply and decrease the complement (*see* p. 52).

If you are told that it is not worth the effort then you can disagree, because you believe that even a little breast-milk is better than none at all and that it is possible to increase the amount.

QUOTE FROM A LETTER
(when the baby was 4 months old)

' You may be interested to hear that the breast-feeding is still going extremely well—in spite of the fact that the hospital told me I wouldn't have enough milk.'

QUOTE FROM ANOTHER REPORT

'. . . They are keen for you to breast-feed in theory, but not in practice. If breast-feeding comes easily to you then they don't bother so much, but if one has problems, they are all for filling him up on cow's milk from a bottle and from a teat. . . . They also won't let you get up at night to feed the baby until your fifth or sixth day —so in the night they get a bottle. . . . They also, when you first start feeding him yourself, make you give a complement feed after he has fed from you—it is useless to argue with them over this as one could become very emotional over it, better just to give a little and keep your cool! '

What can I do if my breasts become engorged?

Engorgement of the breasts is a fairly common occurrence and can be very uncomfortable if not treated properly. It usually occurs within the first 3–5 days after delivery, when it is more likely to be due to the increased blood-supply to the breasts and swelling of the tissues rather than to too much milk. Later, when lactation has been established then it is more likely to be due to too much milk.

The symptoms are unmistakable. You are likely to wake up one morning feeling hot yet shivery. You will feel emotionally fragile—easily upset and weepy. When you take off your bra for washing or feeding, your breasts will feel very heavy, hot, hard, and tender to the touch. They will be enlarged, swollen, and tense—' like lumps of concrete ' was the way one woman described them. The glands under your arms may also be enlarged, and you will probably have a raised temperature and feel very thirsty.

As soon as you have recognized the condition, do the following:—

1. Take your face-cloth and towel and go to the bathroom. Let the cold water tap run, and drape the towel round your waist (to catch any drips). Remove your bra and wet the face-cloth. Squeeze out some of the water but do not wring it too dry. Apply the wet cloth to the upper part of one breast.

   Leave it there for a little while until the cloth feels warm. (You may even see steam rising out of the cloth.) Then cool the cloth again under the cold tap and replace it on the same part of the breast until this part is cool and feels better.

   Give the rest of the breast the same treatment by placing the cold wet cloth on each side of the breast as well as on the lower part of the breast.

   Then treat the other breast in the same way.

   If you do it correctly you will get immediate relief. Do remember that it is not just the surface of the breast that you are treating. You want the cold to seep into the deeper structure of the breast. So it is important to place *at least 2 cold compresses on each part of the engorged breast* for the treatment to be effective. It may be necessary to repeat this treatment several times that day, so do not hesitate to do so and the cold will reduce the swelling.

2. At the same time try to reduce the amount of fluid that you drink. Because you are thirsty you will want to drink a great deal more than usual, but instead drink only half cups of tea or coffee and not the full amount. In between, when you feel thirsty rinse your mouth frequently with cold water and swallow only one or two mouthfuls rather than a full glass.

3. Feed your baby as usual and let him suck from each breast at every feed.

4. Do not express. If the engorgement is due to venous congestion there will be very little to express, and it will be very painful to express from swollen breasts. If the engorgement is due to too much milk then by expressing you are only stimulating the breasts to create more milk, thus perpetuating the engorgement and your discomfort unnecessarily.

5. Keep your breasts well supported day and night by wearing a good supporting bra.

6. Avoid breast exercises which will pump more blood to the breasts.

7. If the breasts are so swollen that the baby cannot grasp the nipple easily, then apply cold compresses before a feed and use a rubber nipple-shield. The baby, by sucking on the nipple-shield, will draw out the nipple and then he can be put directly on to the breast.

Note: It is as well to know that the above treatment, although very effective, is considered unorthodox. Standard hospital treatment (which many women have described as very painful) may include any or all of the following:—

1. Massaging the swollen breasts with warm oil.

2. Hot compresses.

32

3. Expressing—either by hand, breast pump, or electric milking machine.
4. Hormone injections or hormone pills.
5. Binding the breasts tightly.

What should I do if my baby falls asleep after sucking for only 2 minutes?

It is fairly common in the early days for a baby to fall asleep while sucking and before he has taken a full feed. This, however, should not be encouraged, and after a pause lasting no more than 10–15 seconds the baby should be urged to feed again by any of the following means:—

1. Attempt to draw the nipple out of his mouth gently— but do not pull it out. He will then start sucking more vigorously.
2. With your finger press his lower jaw up. This very often is an adequate stimulus to make him suck again.
3. As he begins to doze, undo his blankets and expose his warm tummy to the cooler air. This makes him less warm, comfortable, and snug, and so he wakes up.
4. Change him over to the other breast.

But if you have not been successful, then put him down and let him sleep. He will wake a little later and be more likely to suck properly.

STRUGGLING TO FEED A SLEEPY BABY WILL ONLY FRUSTRATE AND EXHAUST YOU.

If he is so sleepy that he demands less than 5 feeds in 24 hours then it is advisable to have him examined by a doctor.

Note: There is no need—nor is it a good idea—to flick the soles of his feet, sponge his face with cold water, shake him, or use other drastic means to wake him up.

If I bottle-feed in the hospital can I breast-feed when I get home?

Yes, this is possible, as shown in the quotation on p. 9. This is how you effect the change-over. Let your baby suck for a few minutes on each breast at every feed and then give the bottle-feed as a complement. Gradually, taking a week if necessary, increase the sucking time to 10 minutes on each breast and reduce the complement by $\frac{1}{2}$ oz. every 5–7 days.

Work according to your baby's ability to adjust himself to the smaller complement. At the same time work up the milk-supply, as described on p. 52.

Make sure that the hole in the teat is not too large or he will get the bottle-feed too easily and will then be reluctant to suck from the breast.

Should I or should I not burp the baby?

A young baby tends to swallow a fair amount of air while feeding so that his stomach is filled with milk and air. If he is held in the upright position the air (wind), being a gas and lighter than the milk, will rise to the top and come out easily.

But a young baby cannot maintain the upright position because his muscles are not yet strong enough (before he is 6 months old) to support him, and so he tends to sag forward. The resulting pressure on his stomach will force out not only 'wind' but milk also.

So hold him upright and lean him slightly back. Pat his *bottom* gently or stroke his back, but do not wake him up.

If he has not burped within 1–2 minutes, put him down in the crib and let him sleep. The wind will travel down his digestive tract and will come out from the lower end.

You may raise the upper part of his body in the crib by

placing a pillow *under his mattress* (not on top of the mattress, which can be dangerous and might result in suffocation), and then he will burp on his own quite easily while he is lying down.

But if you wake him up by thumping his back to burp him, then you will find it difficult to settle him again, and it will be hardly fair to blame it on 'wind'. It is unpleasant to have one's *upper back* thumped so do not do it to your baby.

Also, avoid pressure on his abdomen or milk will be forced out as well as air.

I am planning to return to work soon after my baby is born. Should I breast-feed for a few weeks and then wean him, or should I not attempt to breast-feed at all but give him bottle-feeds from the time that he is born?

This is a problem which affects not only women who plan to return to work but also women who lead an active social life. Here I would like to stress that breast-feeding can, when necessary, be successfully combined with bottle-feeding. You can breast-feed the baby when you are at home, and when you are away the baby can be given bottle-feeds. Even a small amount of breast-milk is better than none at all for the young baby, and in spite of what women are told it is worth the effort.

Women are often discouraged from continuing with breast-feeding if they have to work, and are told erroneously that breast-milk and formula milk do not mix. On the contrary, breast-feeding and bottle-feeding can be combined very successfully by giving either complementary feeds (bottle-feed after a breast-feed) or supplementary feeds (bottle-feed instead of a breast-feed).

Here are a few examples of how it can be arranged.

EXAMPLE 1

If you are working from 8 a.m. to 5 p.m.

> Early morning feed (±6 a.m.): breast-feed.
> Late morning feed (±10 a.m.): bottle-feed.
> Early afternoon feed (±2 p.m.): bottle-feed.
> Late afternoon feed (±6 p.m.): breast-feed.
> Night feed (between 6 p.m. and 6 a.m.): breast-feed.

The baby will get 2 bottle-feeds and 3 breast-feeds per day, i.e., more than half of his diet consists of breast-milk. At week-ends you will breast-feed only. Do not bother to get the baby used to the bottle before you start working, as he will learn very quickly to drink from the bottle when he is hungry. Also, he may refuse to take a bottle-feed from you because he can smell the breast-milk when you hold him.

EXAMPLE 2

You may be able to change the feeding hours to suit your job. This is how a clinic doctor arranged her feeding schedule so that she could entirely breast-feed and yet do her work and have a social life.

> 8 a.m.: breast-feed.
> 9 a.m.: clinic.
> 12 noon: breast-feed.
> 2 p.m.: clinic.
> 4–4.30 p.m.: breast-feed.
> 8 p.m.: breast-feed.
> Out for the evening.
> ±Midnight: breast-feed.

So, you see that you can arrange breast-feeding to suit yourself and not feel tied down by breast-feeding.

If for some reason it is not possible for you to combine breast-feeding with bottle-feeding, then it will still be better for both you and your baby to start breast-feeding and after a few weeks begin a slow wean. There are three good reasons for doing so, in preference to not attempting to breast-feed at all:—

1. You avoid any risk of thrombosis or embolism as the hormones given to suppress lactation can carry this risk.
2. You avoid the possibility of a breast abscess. If lactation is suddenly suppressed without hormones, a build-up of pressure in the breast may result in an abscess.
3. Your baby gets the benefit of colostrum and breast-milk in the first few weeks of his life when he is most vulnerable.

Should the baby have one bottle-feed a day, so that my husband can participate in feeding him?

No, this is not a good reason for substituting a cow's milk feed for a breast-milk feed. Your husband is involved, but his role as a father is different from yours as a mother, and he can help in many other ways without having to feed the baby.

It would be much better for all of you if you breast-feed happily while your husband keeps you company and observes the baby while he is feeding. After the feed, if your husband wants to, he can take over and put the baby down to sleep and tuck him in.

If for some reason you are very tired or are not feeling well, then your husband can also help by holding the baby to each breast for feeding while you rest or doze.

Only if you have to be away from home for a feed should you leave a bottle-feed for the baby, but when you are at home the baby should be breast-fed.

There is no need to give the baby bottle-feeds in advance 'to get him used to the bottle'. He learns very quickly and if he is hungry he will take the bottle. If, however, the bottle is offered several times and he still refuses to take it, then he will neither starve nor suffer any ill-effects if he waits until you return and can breast-feed him.

If my toddler wants to imitate the baby and also suck at the breast, should I allow it?

Tell your toddler that only babies are fed in this way and that when he was a baby he too was fed from the breast. Now that he is a big boy and has teeth he can eat the same food as grown-ups, like Mum and Dad.

It is not a good idea to let him suck at the breast because he may want to repeat it again, and then it will be more difficult to stop him. Also he may bite you, as by now he will have forgotten how to suck.

How many feeds a day should the baby have?

Young mothers are often encouraged to get their babies on to 3 meals per day as soon as possible. This is considered a great achievement. In actual fact this is quite senseless and should be avoided.

Consider, for example, the number of feedings that the average adult has:—

1. Breakfast.
2. Mid-morning coffee.
3. Lunch.
4. Afternoon tea.
5. Evening meal (supper, dinner, or high tea).
6. A snack later in the evening, e.g., after a show, or if entertaining friends at home, or visiting friends, or even a warm drink while watching TV at home.

Now adults are no longer growing in height—they can only grow sideways—and yet they have 6 feedings in 24 hours, whereas a young baby, who needs food for growth and development, and has a small capacity, is restricted to 3 feedings in the 24 hours.

If what the baby requires for the 24 hours were to be given in 3 feeds instead of 5 or 6 feeds, then one of two things is likely to happen:—

1. He will reject some of the feed because he cannot accommodate the extra amount and so will not get what he needs, and also he will develop a bad habit of vomiting.

2. His stomach will gradually 'stretch' to hold a larger volume of liquid than he needs at this stage of development, so that in future he will always want more food to fill his stomach than he needs.

It is true that it is the bottle-fed baby who is at greater risk of being given only 3 huge feeds per day, but unless the mother who is breast-feeding her baby is aware that this is not desirable she may feel that she is incapable of giving her baby enough breast-milk or that her baby is not progressing as quickly as the bottle-fed baby, and she may decide to give up breast-feeding in favour of bottle-feeding.

Whether the baby is being breast-fed or bottle-fed it is better for him to have small feeds every 3 or 4 hours, i.e., 5–6 feeds in the 24 hours, rather than 3 large feeds. If the milk-supply is inadequate and the baby wants even more frequent feeds for a short spell, then this is quite normal and permissible and far better than giving 3 feeds with complements of artificial feeds.

A young baby needs to be fed:—

> Early in the morning: about 6 a.m.
> Late in the morning: about 10 a.m.
> Early in the afternoon: about 2 p.m.
> Late in the afternoon: about 6 p.m.
> During the night: between 6 p.m. and 6 a.m.

Babies may vary in their feeding patterns. Some babies demand 2 feeds during the night, i.e., between 6 p.m. and 6 a.m., and this is perfectly normal for the first 3 months. Some babies want frequent day feeds—about 3-hourly—but will sleep for a long spell at night, i.e., 6 p.m. to 6 a.m. This, too, is normal, because the baby gets 5 feeds in 24 hours.

My baby now sleeps through the night, and so gets only 4 feeds per day. Should I wake him for an extra feed?
Although most babies require 5 feeds per day until they are 7–8 months old, there are exceptions. Also most babies do not like to be woken as they get older. They get fractious and irritable, they do not feed well, and they will not settle afterwards, and, of course, the whole family is then disturbed.

So what you do will depend on your individual baby.

IF HE IS GAINING WELL OR IS
SLIGHTLY OVERWEIGHT
1. It is better not to wake him. Let him have 4 feeds only, and after a while you may find that he is demanding an extra feed. In which case give it to him. But if he continues to gain and is happy on 4 feeds, then just leave him.
2. If he is over 4 months old check the amount of solids he is taking, and if necessary reduce the helpings. Your guide is:—

> 4–6 months: 1 flat tablespoon of any solid food.
> 6–9 months: 1–2 flat tablespoons of any solid food.

IF HE IS GAINING SLOWLY OR IS
SLIGHTLY UNDERWEIGHT
1. Try to fit in an extra feed during the day, or feed him

3-hourly in the daytime. Some babies prefer frequent day feeds and then sleep through the night.

2. You may be able to give him a night-feed without waking him. Pick him up gently and put him to the breast. He will suck without waking and will carry on sleeping when tucked in again. (Do not change his nappy or he will wake up. It is assumed that he does not wear plastic pants, which of course predispose to nappy rash.)

3. He may be the exception. In which case he will be quite happy to be woken and fed before you go to bed.

My baby at 5 months is quite happy on 3 feeds per day. What shall I do?

In general it is better for a baby to have several small, frequent feeds rather than 3 large feeds per day. (*See* p. 38).

You may find that by reducing the sucking time on each breast he will get less per feed.

Also, make quite sure that you do not give more than one *flat* tablespoon of any of his solid foods.

In this way, by reducing the size of each feed, he will, after a day or two, require an extra feed.

My baby used to sleep through the night, but now he wakes. Should I feed him?

It may not necessarily be hunger that wakes your baby during the night. There are many other reasons why a baby wakes at night. For example, he may be cold, either because the temperature in the room has dropped or because he has a wet nappy and has kicked off the bedclothes. He may have a tummy-ache or an ear-ache, or he may even have had a bad dream and feels insecure or frightened.

If, however, you have eliminated other causes and feel that he is hungry, then put him to the breast and feed him without any feelings of annoyance, resentment, or guilt. If he is over 8 months old then also increase the amount of protein he has for supper. The extra protein will enable him to sleep longer.

Although my baby is gaining weight he is not happy. He cries all the time. Should I change to bottle-feeding?

It is not the breast-milk that makes him cry, so if you change to bottle-feeding he will still cry. Then you will increase the size of the feed, and if that does not solve your problem—as it will not—you will increase the strength of the feed, and this will create other problems, including a weight problem, tummy cramps, constipation, and sour-smelling regurgitations.

If the baby is gaining weight and his stools are normal (daffodil yellow in colour) and he is not vomiting, then you can be reassured that the cause of his trouble is not feeding, but rather it is your handling of the baby which is at fault.

To correct this try the following suggestions:—

1. When the baby wakes and cries out, go to him *immediately*.

2. Talk to him happily and cheerfully, and smile at him while you pick him up, change his nappy, prepare the crib, and get ready to feed him. This is done to attract his attention and to stimulate his interest, and if you are successful it will stop him crying. Also, in this way you will calm yourself as well as the baby.

3. While you feed him make sure that you are quite relaxed. Check your shoulders, wrists, and fingers for

unnecessary tension. You will find that if you are relaxed it will rub off on the baby and he, too, will be more relaxed. You will be able to judge this for yourself if you observe the baby's hands. If his fists are tightly clenched then he is tense and insecure. But if his hands are relaxed then he, too, is relaxed and happy.

4. Encourage him to fall asleep towards the end of the feed.

5. Do not wake him up to burp him, but place him in his crib on his side, tuck him up, and make sure that a fold of blanket covers his ear.

6. If he stirs make gentle soporific sounds (Shhhh . . . shhhh . . . etc.). At the same time place one hand firmly over his shoulder and pat his bottom with the other hand firmly and slowly. If he cries pat harder. If he stops crying make the patting gradually lighter but continue until he has fallen asleep. Then slowly release the pressure on his shoulder. Rhythmic movements are very comforting and soothing, but if you stop suddenly or too soon he will jerk awake.

Note: A baby is very sensitive to the emotional climate around him, so do not feel sorry for him. Instead, tell him that he is the luckiest baby in the world—he has loving parents, a good home, the best possible food, grandparents, cousins, uncles, aunts—and anything else you wish to add. But do beware of pity or he will feel sorry for himself and continue to cry.

If the baby is not gaining weight, does this indicate the need to change to bottle-feeding?

A baby has to grow, and the increase in weight is an important index of his growth. At the same time if he is not gaining, other factors have to be considered. So do not give up breast-feeding but consider the following:—

1. Make sure that he is perfectly fit and well, because some babies do not gain weight if they are ill or fretting. (Babies in institutions sometimes fail to thrive even though they get adequate nourishment.) If you have any doubts at all about his health, let your doctor or the clinic doctor give him a complete check-up.

2. Assess his weight in relation to his age (*see* p. 61), and if he is slightly overweight then do not worry. He can afford to be stationary in weight for a few weeks. This often happens if the baby is getting only 4 feeds in 24 hours (instead of 5 or 6 feeds) even though he has previously gained on 4 feeds.

3. If he is the correct weight for his age, or slightly underweight, then try to fit in 1 or 2 extra breast-feeds during the day. It may be possible to feed him 3-hourly instead of 4-hourly for a few weeks, or you can pick him up (without waking him) and give him an extra feed before you go to bed. Most babies will suck quite happily even though they are half asleep. But do not try to change his nappy and do not burp him or you will wake him up, and then you may have difficulty in settling him.

4. If you have doubts about your milk-supply, then increase the amount (*see* p. 52).

5. It is better to give the baby as much breast-milk as you have and a small complement, if necessary, after each breast-feed, than to change completely to bottle-feeding. When he starts gaining again you can then gradually reduce the complement until he is once more wholly breast-fed, or he can continue with the small complement.

44

6. The baby should also be considered as an individual and not as an automatic machine. A little girl who is well and happy and has a small appetite should not be stuffed with extra food just to put on more weight. She may be the *petite* and dainty type and it would be sad to turn her into a fat pudding.

7. Remember that most babies do not gain weight in the week after they have been immunized or vaccinated.

Why doesn't my baby settle after feeds?

There may be several reasons for this:—

1. The baby may still be hungry, especially if he is not gaining weight.

What to do

a. Give him a small complement: 1 oz. boiled cow's milk plus 1 oz. boiled water. There is no need for sugar as it is a temporary measure. Let him have what he wants but do not urge him to take it all.

b. Work up your milk-supply (*see* p. 52).

2. The baby may have a tummy-ache from too much food.

What to do

Apply warmth to his tummy. Fold two gauze nappies into small rectangles and iron one on both sides. Check to make sure that it is not too hot and place it on baby's tummy. Now warm the other nappy by ironing it on both sides. Check that this one, too, is not too hot and apply to the baby's tummy, removing the first nappy, which you now warm again. Continue to replace the cooled pads by warm ones until the baby is more comfortable. You may have to iron *each pad* five or six times, but this is a very effective method for treating a tummy-ache.

3. The baby may feel insecure because you are anxious, worried, or just unsure of yourself.

What to do

Relax and sing him a lullaby. Pat his bottom, or wheel him up and down.

4. The baby is woken up after the feed to have his nappy changed.

What to do

Change his nappy before the feed rather than after. Even if he wets it again while feeding there are no irritating substances in his urine or stool to cause nappy rash, and his nervous system is too immature for him to be aware of the wet nappy as long as it is warm.

5. By far the most common reason is patting the baby vigorously on his back to burp him. A baby who is getting enough breast-milk tends to become sleepy towards the end of his feed, and this state should be encouraged. But very often by patting his back to burp him the mother wakes him up, and after that she is surprised that he will not settle and go to sleep again.

What to do

Let the baby fall asleep while feeding him and then hold him upright and leaning slightly back and he will burp without waking. You may even pat his bottom (not his upper back) or gently rub his back without waking him. If you place a pillow under his mattress, thus slightly raising the upper part of his body, he will burp on his own. And if he does not then it will come out of the other end.

6. Some mothers believe that they should 'mother' the baby by playing with him after feeds. This is a great mistake because the longer the baby is kept awake after a feed the more difficult it is to settle him afterwards.

What to do

Play and talk to him before feeds while you change his nappy and get yourself ready. Encourage him to be sleepy towards the end of the feed.

7. A difficult time very often is after the 6 p.m. feed when you are tired. You may not even be aware of your tiredness then, but it is only to be expected if you have been awake since 5 or 6 a.m. for the baby's first feed of the day.

Also you may, without realizing it, be rather urgent and anxious about wanting to settle the baby quickly so that you can prepare the evening meal and be ready when your husband comes home. You may even, when you are feeding the baby, be thinking about the cooking.

The baby senses all this and reacts to the general unsettled atmosphere and your tiredness by feeling insecure, and so will not settle.

Because you are unaware of your tiredness and urgency and cannot find any logical reason for his restlessness, you will tend to worry about the amount of breast-milk he is getting and whether he is still hungry, or you may even attribute his behaviour to '3 months colic'.

What to do

If you have tried all the suggestions on p. 48 without success, then prop him up in his crib, pram, or relaxing chair (if he has one) and position him where he can watch you.

Make sure that he is snugly wrapped up so that he feels more secure. Turn on the radio or television sound or sing to him while you prepare the evening meal, set the table, etc.

As soon as you see him squirm and sense that he is about to cry, attract his attention by talking to him. When you talk to your baby talk naturally like you would to an adult, calmly and deliberately. Aim to keep his attention, and do not make it a dull monotonous monologue.

In this way you can keep him quiet for quite some time. After a while, when you sense that he is getting irritable and tired, pick him up, change his nappy, and offer him each breast again. You will find then that he will settle more easily afterwards.

Note: Never leave the baby to cry. His cry is a call to you and you should not ignore it. Crying will not resolve any problem but is likely to exhaust the baby and make him more and more panic-stricken. It may also lead to nervy and whining behaviour later.

In general, to help your baby to settle after feeds you will find the following suggestions helpful:—

1. Aim for the feed to be quiet, peaceful, and conducive to dozing off. Make sure that you are relaxed—not only your body but your mind, too. Do not anticipate any difficulties.
2. Encourage him to fall asleep while sucking on the second breast.
3. If he is still wide awake let him suck for another few minutes on each breast, if the nipples are not tender.
4. Do not bang his back after a feed to burp him. It will jerk him awake and then he will not settle.
5. Place a hot-water bottle in his crib *before* you start feeding and *remove it* as you lay him down after the feed, so that he lies on a warm area. This is very soothing. (Never leave a hot-water bottle with a baby because of the risk of burns.)
6. When he is on his side and tucked in, place a fold of

blanket over his upper ear and the back of his head. This helps to make him feel more snug. In summer, use a gauze nappy instead of a fold of blanket.

7. Patting his bottom, rocking the cradle, or wheeling him up and down may also help him to fall asleep after feeds.

8. You may, if you wish and as a last resort, let him suck a dummy to help him fall asleep. Use the dummy as a crutch only—a temporary aid until he has learned to go to sleep after feeds. Do not use it indiscriminately as a means of keeping him quiet.

What can I do if the milk comes too quickly and the baby seems to choke?

This can be a problem in the early weeks of breast-feeding, and although it is only a temporary problem it can be distressing both for the mother and the baby unless it is handled properly.

The common mistake is to let the baby come off the breast. He then continues to splutter and choke and gets panicky and distressed. To prevent this happening hold the baby's head firmly so that he cannot come off the breast.

He will then have to take a few large swallows and will also have to breathe through his nose. In this way choking is avoided. At the same time reassure him with your voice.

What can be done when the baby gets hiccups?

This is a common occurrence among young babies and, although the babies are not upset by the hiccups, their mothers tend to worry unduly about them.

Hiccups are caused by spasms of the diaphragm, and

the best and quickest way to stop them is to put the baby to the breast for a few minutes. Making the baby suck stops the hiccups quite dramatically.

Why do I get cramps in my tummy when I feed the baby?
The hormone oxytocin, which is released when the baby sucks, also contracts the muscle of the uterus (womb). Some women are aware of this as tummy cramps when they breast-feed in the early weeks and until the uterus has shrunk back to its normal size. Other women notice that the lochia (vaginal discharge after the baby's birth) increases slightly when they breast-feed. But these things happen because breast-feeding is helping your internal organs to return to their normal state more quickly and completely than if you were bottle-feeding.

Why does my baby struggle when he feeds?
Observe him carefully and decide which one of the following possibilities is responsible:—
1. If there is an abundance of milk and he cannot swallow it quickly enough it may give the impression that he is struggling.
What to do
Reassure him while he feeds and the condition will settle down within a day or two. If necessary reduce the milk-supply (*see* p. 60).
2. If he gets what he needs in a few minutes and you try to make him suck for the full 10 minutes on each breast he may react by struggling.
What to do
Do not force him. Let him take what he wants.
3. If he is not getting enough milk his behaviour may also give the impression of struggling. Here his behaviour

is very characteristic: he gives a few sucks, pulls away, arching his back, lets go the nipple and yells, grabs at the nipple again, and repeats the performance again and again. You will also be able to sense his frustration at sucking and getting virtually no milk.

What to do

Give him a complement of equal amounts of boiled cow's milk and boiled water, and increase your milk-supply (*see* p. 52).

4. If the mother is tired, worried, or upset the baby may react to her state and not feed calmly.

What to do

Try to relax while you feed and calm yourself by breathing very slowly and deeply for a while. Reassure the baby with soft soothing sounds.

5. Some babies, when over-tired and over-wrought, struggle at the breast.

What to do

Rock him in your arms and calm him down before putting him to the breast. If necessary, pat his bottom while he feeds. Try not to let him get into such a state again.

6. A baby who has become accustomed to bottle-feeding may refuse to suck properly at the breast and appears to struggle to get away.

What to do

Calm yourself and the baby and offer the other breast, and alternate from breast to breast for a while. A little honey or breast-milk on the nipple may help him to take it. Rhythmic patting while holding him to the breast will also help. Sometimes if you hold him to the breast at a different angle from the usual one he will feed quite well, e.g., with his legs directed towards your back instead of sitting on your lap.

7. Some babies do not feed well if they have a full bowel and have difficulty in emptying it.

What to do

You may start giving him the juice of stewed prunes and later, if necessary, give the prune pulp as well. Start with a little and gradually work up the amount until the baby no longer fusses and his bowel empties easily.

What can I do if I do not have enough breast-milk?

Be assured that the milk-supply can be increased and that there is no magic involved.

Many cases have been reported where women who had not recently been pregnant had put adopted babies to the breast and had worked up an adequate supply of breast-milk.

In Central Africa many young mothers have to leave their babies in the care of grandparents while they have to go away to work in the towns. Often the grandmother will put the baby to her breast and within a short time be completely breast-feeding her grandchild.

And if grandmothers and foster mothers who have not recently produced babies can do it, then think how much better equipped you are to do it. Suckling is the most powerful means of stimulating breast activity. So here is what you have to do:—

1. Feed the baby frequently on both breasts. The interval between feeds can be 2 hours, or even 1½ hours. But do not let the baby suck for more than 10 minutes on each breast. This is to prevent tender nipples. The sucking will stimulate the release of oxytocin, which in turn liberates prolactin.

2. Practise physical relaxation several times a day, especially before feeds, and make sure that while you are feeding you are relaxed—check on shoulders, arms, wrists, and fingers, and relax the muscles of your face. Smile at your baby.

Breathing slowly will help, expecially breathing out. Emotions like anxiety, doubt, worry, indecision, etc. interfere with the normal internal functioning of the body. But if you are relaxed then you cannot at the same time feel these negative emotions.

A good cry very often helps to release tension.

3. Increase your fluid intake. Drink 1–2 glasses of water while feeding and 1–2 cups of fluid between feeds. This is as a rule no problem, as women tend to be naturally more thirsty than usual in the early weeks of breast-feeding. But do not force yourself to drink or the emotional strain and urgency involved may actually inhibit milk production. Be casual and intelligent about the matter.

4. Avoid coffee temporarily as it has an inhibiting effect on the production of milk.

5. Alcohol prevents the release of oxytocin. So avoid alcoholic drinks for a while.

6. Vitamin B works wonders. Take it in the form of D.C.L. tablets or pure brewer's yeast tablets: 2–3 tablets 3 times per day after meals. (Chew them if you can.)

7. Vitamin E (100 mg. per day) is also helpful.

8. After feeds spend 20–30 seconds doing a simple exercise. Grasp your wrists, raise elbows to shoulder level, and push the skin of the lower arms smartly towards the elbows. An alternative exercise is to gently swing each arm in turn in a wide circle—forward, up, back,

and down. These exercises help to increase the blood circulation to the breasts.

9. There is no need to drink milk. Cow's milk does not make breast-milk, and you do run the risk of putting on weight if you drink milk in addition to your normal well-balanced and well-mixed diet.

10. There is a nasal spray (Syntocinon) on the market which aids the let-down reflex. This would have to be prescribed by your doctor, but it is rarely necessary as the simple suggestions described above are, as a rule, quite adequate.

Note: If you are able to lie down and rest for a while, then it is sensible to have the baby in his crib, carry-cot, or pram next to you, so that if he stirs you can soothe him by rocking or patting him, and if he is sleeping peacefully you do not have to get anxious and to worry why he is so quiet, or to rush to see him to make sure that he is still alive and breathing.

Why is my baby suddenly refusing to feed even though my breasts are full?

This is not a very common problem, but when it occurs it is very sudden and unexpected, and the baby will be at least 2 months old.

The baby, who has previously fed very well, begins to cry when an attempt is made to feed him. He will lie happily in his mother's lap and smile and coo at her, but as soon as she attempts to feed him he struggles, cries, and refuses even to take the nipple in his mouth. Left alone he seems quite happy (although some babies are a bit grissly at this time), but feed he will not. It is almost as if he has gone on a hunger strike.

The reason for this strange behaviour seems to be

54

associated with the mother's menstrual cycle—either the onset of menstruation or her pre-menstrual tension to which the baby reacts. It is thought that at this time the familiar smell of either the breast-milk or the mother is slightly different.

What to do

1. Do accept and believe that your baby will not starve if he misses one or two feeds.
2. Reassure him when he cries by talking to him softly, slowly, and soothingly.
3. Do not force him to take the breast while he is screaming and struggling. It will only make things worse.
4. Do not give him a bottle-feed as an alternative.
5. Have a warm bath which has been liberally scented with some bath perfume. Laze in it and relax. In summer you may prefer a cool scented bath. This is to mask the unfamiliar smell to which the baby is reacting.
6. Offer him the breast immediately after the bath and you will probably find that he will feed quite well then. This works almost magically.
7. Be prepared to have several scented leisurely baths in one day.
8. However, if he is very obstinate then persevere by offering the breast when a feed is due, or when he appears to be hungry. Do so calmly and lovingly. If he still refuses to feed, comfort him and leave him. Do *not* give him a bottle-feed. By the end of the day he will have got used to the unfamiliar smell and will be sufficiently hungry to take the breast.
9. Sometimes applying expressed milk or honey to the nipple will encourage the baby to feed again.
10. The baby may behave in this way for a day or two. But the more positive you are in handling him the

more quickly he will settle down and feed normally.

11. Do not be surprised or upset if the same performance happens a month later. Persevere as suggested above and you will find that the baby's reaction and behaviour improves each time.

My baby has a preference for one breast. How can I correct it?

1. Offer the non-favourite breast first at every feed and encourage your baby to suck for as long as possible—but not much longer than 10 minutes.
2. Build up the milk-supply so that he gets the milk easily and does not have to struggle at the breast.
3. You may have to hold him at a different angle for him to feed from that breast, e.g., hold him between your arm and body and support his head with your hand.
4. Try not to anticipate any trouble before each feed. Be relaxed when feeding, but also be firm. Babies are influenced by the mother's emotional state and if you are confident about what you are doing he will respond.
5. Sometimes it helps to pat his bottom while you are trying to get him to take the breast. Any rhythmic movement is comforting and reassuring for the young baby.
6. He may be tempted to suck if he tastes a little expressed breast-milk or honey on the nipple.

Note: Generally, with a little perseverance the problem can be corrected. But if not, then be assured that it is still possible to breast-feed from only one breast.

My baby seems hungry. Can I give him cereal?

If your baby is hungry then he needs milk, not cereal. Milk forms the most important part of his diet in the first

9 months of his life. It is a poor exchange, therefore, to give cereal, which is a starch, instead of milk, which is a protein food.

So, if your baby seems hungry, fill a feeding bottle with a mixture of 4 oz. of boiled cow's milk and 4 oz. of boiled water. Let him take as much as he wants, but do not urge him to finish it all. From now on aim to work up your supply of breast-milk (*see* p. 52).

The reasons for giving cereal after the baby is 4 months old is *not* to supplement his diet but to *teach* him:—
1. To eat off a spoon.
2. To eat semi-solid food, i.e., a different consistency to the fluid of milk.
3. To accept different tastes.

Cereal should be one item of a mixed diet but it should never be considered as the most important item. Babies who are overweight should be given very little cereal and only once a day. It may even be omitted altogether and fruit given instead because cereal will increase a baby's weight, just as starchy foods will make an adult put on weight. And it is not good for either babies or adults to be fat and overweight.

My baby screams and screams until he is fed. Is he greedy?
Poor little babies, who cannot defend themselves, have often been maligned and labelled greedy by adults who do not understand them. But it is panic and not greed which is the cause of his frantic behaviour, and unless you deal with it promptly and properly it may become a habit, as will your solution of always pacifying him with food.

Just because he has to stop crying while he feeds does not necessarily mean that the cause was hunger. A baby is getting enough food if he has 5 feeds in 24 hours, is gaining weight, and has yellow stools (the shade of yellow has been likened to gold, mustard, or daffodils).

So, when he wakes and screams for his feed, go to him immediately. Pick him up and hold him tightly and close to your body (to calm him down). Shush him by talking to him with confidence and conviction, e.g., ' quiet! quiet! I love you dearly, but stop crying! ' etc., and reinforce every word with a firm pat on his bottom (not his back).

Babies are very sensitive to the emotional atmosphere around them, and the more confident you are about what you are doing and why you are doing it the more effective it will be. Conversely, the more frantic his behaviour the more upset you become. The more upset you are the more insecure the baby feels and the more he yells.

It is up to you to break this vicious circle. Only you can do it. We cannot rely on or expect the baby to do it. When the baby has quietened down, change his nappy and feed him. A baby learns from what is done to him, and in this way he will learn that there is no need for him to scream in panic and that he will be fed only when he is calm. Whereas if you constantly offer him the breast when he screams, then he will expect to be fed every time he screams, and may even consider the feed a reward for screaming.

Do not be discouraged if at your first attempt you are not sufficiently confident to be completely successful, and you may even find that once or twice you have to give the breast before he is quiet. But if you know what to aim for, and you persevere, then you will both learn.

Even if you are convinced that he is 'greedy', do not encourage this frantic behaviour, or the 'greed'. A baby has to be guided to behave in a way which will be to his benefit not only now but also in the future.

Can you overfeed on breast-milk only?

A baby can be overfed on breast-milk as well as on any other food. If the amount of food taken in is more than his body requires, all the extra nourishment which he swallows will be stored as fat (to be utilized in lean times of food shortage). Fat is hard and solid, so do not be misled and lulled into smug complacency by the fact that the baby is 'fat and firm' and not 'fat and flabby', as you have been led to expect.

Early signs of overfeeding on breast-milk include:—
1. Constantly spitting up some milk after feeds.
2. Frequent bright-green frothy stools, or yellow stools tinged with bright-green.
3. Abdominal discomfort and tummy cramps, resulting in crying and fretfulness.
4. The weekly weight-gain will exceed 8 oz. (To be judged over a period of several weeks.)
5. His weight will be more than that recommended for his age. (*See* chart on p. 61.)

What to do

As a temporary measure reduce the time of sucking at each breast by a few minutes, or reduce the number of feeds to 4 per day. (If he has been getting 6 feeds per day, reduce the number to 5).

After a few weeks when the problem has been corrected you can gradually increase the length of feeds again, because by then the baby will be older and will need and be able to cope with larger feeds.

What if I have too much milk? How can I reduce the amount?

During the puerperium (the first 6–8 weeks after birth) the milk-supply can be rather erratic, but very soon it settles down and from then on the amount of breast-milk that you secrete will depend to a large extent on the amount of stimulation that the breasts receive. If, however, you still have too much milk then you can reduce the amount as follows:—

1. Gradually reduce the baby's sucking time at each breast from 10 minutes to as little as 5 minutes if necessary. This will reduce the stimulation to the breasts.

2. Even though you may feel very thirsty, try to *reduce* the amount of fluid that you drink (but do not cut out all fluids).

3. No matter how uncomfortable the breasts feel, do not express any milk from them. Instead, apply frequent cold compresses to your breasts (*see* p. 31).

4. Avoid any breast exercises (which will increase the blood-supply to your breasts).

5. It may be necessary to let your baby suck from one breast only at each feed, so that each breast is stimulated less frequently. In this way, within a day or two, the milk-supply will be reduced.

How can I prevent my baby becoming too fat?

To be overweight is to be at a grave disadvantage in life, and far too often the seeds of obesity are sown in infancy. So aim to prevent it as follows:—

1. Know what is the desired weight for the baby as he grows. Use the following table as your guide, allowing a margin of about 1 lb. either way.

Age (Months)	Weight (lb.)
Birth	6–8
1	8–9½
2	10–11
3	12
4	13
5	14
6	15
7	16
8	17
9	18
10	19
11	20
12	21

2. Knowing that your baby at 1 year should be about 20 lb. if a girl, and not more than 22 lb. if a boy, you can work out the desired average weekly or monthly gain according to the baby's birth-weight and sex.

For example: if a baby girl weighs 10 lb. at birth, then she should not be allowed to gain more than about 11 lb. in her first year, i.e., less than 1 lb. per month.

If a baby weighs 5 lb. at birth then he has to gain about 16 lb. in his first year, i.e., about 5 oz. per week.

3. Bear in mind that babies tend to put on weight more rapidly in the first few months of life, and then the weight-gain slows down. So do not worry unduly if he is gaining more than he should for a few weeks, but do not let this pattern persist.

4. If the baby is constantly gaining too much and his weight is creeping above what it should be, then check his feeding. Try to give him no more than 5 feeds in 24 hours, or it may be possible to reduce his sucking time at each breast by a few minutes.

Remember that you can overfeed on breast-milk as well as on any other kind of food.

5. There is less risk of overweight if a baby is fed according to his age rather than to his weight. So do not

introduce solids before the baby is 4 months old, and when that stage comes give sugar very sparingly and be careful not to stimulate an appetite for sweet foods. Do not let anyone persuade you that ' he is a big baby and therefore needs more food ', or otherwise you will have a grossly overweight baby on your hands before long.

6. If your baby is gaining weight resist the temptation to pacify him everytime he cries or is unhappy and fretful by giving him an extra feed. If this happens often enough he will learn that food will console and comfort him, and this may lead to compulsive eating later on. There are other ways of comforting a fretful baby besides giving food, and it is not always food that he wants, but love, warmth, security, and a feeling of *being safe*.

How can I breast-feed when my baby has teeth? Surely he will bite me?

The mechanism of sucking does not involve gripping the nipple with the gums nor, therefore, with the teeth. So the eruption of teeth does not normally present a problem nor is it a reason for weaning.

You must, however, be aware that the baby is likely to try a tentative bite and *will watch you closely for permission to do it*. If you deter him at this stage, by looking stern and saying ' No! ' firmly and with conviction, then he will never bite you.

But very often the mother, unaware of the significance of the act, smiles reassuringly and does not realize that by so doing she does, in fact, show her approval and gives her baby permission to do it again on some future occasion. As a mother you must be one step ahead of your baby and try to deter or prevent him from starting a bad habit.

Perhaps relating the story of Lisa will help to illustrate the point.

Lisa arrived after her parents had been married for 6 years and had almost given up hope of having a baby. So it is understandable that she was an extra-precious baby. At 6 months she was still being breast-fed and already had several teeth. One Monday morning I had a phone call from Lisa's mother. She was upset and wanted to see me urgently. This is what she told me.

The previous day at the 2 p.m. feed Lisa bit her. This was such a shock to the mother that she reacted instinctively and hit the baby on the leg. Lisa had never before had such treatment and screamed. Being Sunday, Dad was at home and came dashing into the room.

' What on earth is the matter? ' he demanded.

The mother, in tears and feeling ashamed and guilty, as well as suffering from the physical hurt of sharp little teeth on a tender nipple, blurted out:

' I've hit the baby. I've hit the baby. Now you can tell all our friends that I've hit the baby.'

He, not understanding the reason nor the circumstances, reacted with anger and annoyance to her, and concern for the baby, which made the mother feel even worse.

After hearing her story, I reassured the mother that her instinctive response would not be permanently damaging to Lisa, and it would act as a sufficient deterrent in the future. And then I questioned her about a previous practice attempt at biting.

She thought for a while, and then light dawned.

' Oh, yes ', she remembered. ' But I thought how clever of her to know what her teeth were for.'

Without realizing it she had smiled encouragement and had given Lisa the ' go-ahead ' to do it again.

Lisa never bit her mother again and was breast-fed for 9 months.

For how long should breast-feeding continue?

Milk is an almost perfect food, and is the substance that nourishes all young mammals in infancy. For the human baby, milk forms the main item of diet for the first 9 months of life. By then he has some teeth and his digestive system has sufficiently matured to enable him to digest, absorb, and therefore benefit from other foods. Milk then is no longer so important and this indicates that it is time to wean.

Nine months of breast-feeding may seem a very long time, but you will find that once lactation has been established (and sometimes it takes the whole duration of the puerperium to establish lactation) the whole process works so efficiently that it gets easier and takes less time as the baby gets older.

In the early weeks of his life the baby sucks laboriously for 10 minutes on each breast. But as he grows his suction becomes so much stronger that he can get more milk in less time, and his sucking time at the breast tends to decrease.

Some babies at 6 months get all that they need in 3–4 minutes' sucking on each breast, and by 9 months 2–3 minutes on each breast will provide a baby with sufficient milk. Also, his need for sucking decreases as he gets older. (The very young baby is easily comforted by sucking, and it is a source of great emotional satisfaction for him.) Most women enjoy breast-feeding so much that they feel quite sad when the weaning stage comes.

Note: Although breast-milk forms the most important part of the baby's diet for the first 9 months of his life, when he is 1 month old vitamin C and vitamins $A+D$ are given in addition.

Before the baby is 4 months old he lacks the various enzymes which are necessary for the digestion and absorption of other foods. So only when he is 4 months old is a small amount of semi-solid food introduced.

From then on a new food is given every week (starting on the day of the week that the baby was born, as a weekly birthday celebration). And in this way his diet is gradually built up, so that by the time he is 9 months old he is having the same diet as his parents, and like his parents is having 3 meals per day.*

How do I wean the baby off the breast?

At 8 *months* the baby is having a fair amount of ordinary food in addition to his breast-feeds.

The first step in weaning him off the breast is to omit the night feed. This is achieved by giving him extra protein food at the 6 p.m. feed (to enable him to sleep longer). From now on the baby will get only 4 feeds per day.

When he is 9 *months old* cut out another feed by changing over to 3 meals per day. This is done by omitting the early morning breast-feed and giving him his full breakfast at about 7 a.m. As a rule this is easy, but should he wake early and be unhappy and fretful then let him have his fruit juice when he wakes, and give him his

* This subject is dealt with in greater detail in the author's *The Know-how of Infant Feeding.*

breakfast at 7 a.m. His lunch will be at about 1 p.m. and his supper about 6 p.m. Thus, he is now getting 3 meals per day and a breast-feed after each meal.

A week later, when he has adjusted to the new routine, give him a cup-feed of 3 oz. boiled cow's milk with 3 oz. boiled water after his lunch instead of the breast-feed.

It may take a week, or even longer, for him to accept the cup-feed. But persevere, and give him the comfort of the breast after his breakfast and after his supper.

The following week, when he is accepting some milk from the cup, make the next change and give him another cup-feed after his supper. This leaves him with only 1 breast-feed: after breakfast.

The next week, replace this final breast-feed by giving a cup-feed after his breakfast.

Under 8 *months of age* the baby still needs 5 feeds per day and should be weaned on to a bottle. This is indicated by the fact that the sucking pads inside his cheeks only begin to atrophy at about 9 months of age.

Always wean slowly, taking at least 1 week over every change, and cut out feeds alternately. This is to allow the breasts to settle down evenly and naturally, because with less stimulation they will secrete less milk. Also it gives the baby time to adapt to bottle-feeds, and he is not suddenly and completely deprived of the comfort and security of the breast.

Sometimes, if the baby does not adjust easily, it may be necessary to take 10–14 days over each change.

Proceed as follows:—

1*st Week*

Substitute a bottle-feed containing a mixture of 3½ oz. boiled cow's milk and 3½ oz. boiled water after the

10 a.m. or 6 p.m. feed, whichever one you wish. But give him the breast at the other 4 feeds.

2nd Week

Give bottle-feeds at 10 a.m. and 6 p.m. and give breast-feeds at 6 a.m., 2 p.m., and late at night (10–11 p.m.).

3rd Week

Give bottle-feeds at 10 a.m., 2 p.m., and 6 p.m., and give breast-feeds at 6 a.m. and 11 p.m.

4th Week

Give the breast at 6 a.m. only and give 4 bottle-feeds: at 10 a.m., 2 p.m., 6 p.m., and 11 p.m.

5th Week

Bottle-feeds only.

Some babies may be reluctant to give up the breast and will at first refuse to take bottle- or cup-feeds, especially if they can smell the breast-milk. It may then be kinder to let someone else give him the cup- or bottle-feed. Also, babies seldom take the full amount of formula from the bottle or cup, and as a rule they do not gain weight while being weaned.

What must I do if my baby vomits?

The reason for vomiting may vary from something as simple as careless handling (like jogging him after a feed) to some serious illness. So do not ignore it and do not allow it to become a habit. From the following list, and by a process of elimination, find and correct the cause:—

1. A mouthful of milk forced out by a burp after a feed can safely be ignored.

2. *Direct pressure on the abdomen* will result in vomiting. This includes sleeping or lying on his tummy, holding him against your shoulder for burping, allowing him to sit up and sag forward, pressing with a hand on his

tummy, or even dressing him in tight restrictive clothing. With a little care and forethought this type of vomiting can easily be prevented.

3. *Overloading his stomach.* It is always better to give a baby feeds which do not result in vomiting. So do not urge him to take larger feeds than he can hold. If sucking for 10 minutes on each breast results in vomiting, then reduce the time of sucking to 8, 7, or even 6 minutes on each breast. Do remember that most of the feed is taken in the first 4–5 minutes on each breast.

4. *Projectile vomiting.* This means forceful vomiting that shoots out and lands a considerable distance away from the baby. It may be due to either a spasm or an obstruction of the lower part of the stomach (pylorus).

   a. Pyloric spasm is indicated if the baby has projectile vomiting but is passing normal stools. This vomiting can be prevented by letting the baby suck for only 2–3 minutes on each breast every 2 hours. The smaller volume of milk will not be enough to stimulate the spasm. It may take 2–3 weeks for the baby to outgrow this condition. However, if you cannot stop the vomiting this way then consult your doctor who will prescribe antispasmodic medicine.

   b. Pyloric stenosis. If the baby has projectile vomiting and *is not passing stools*, then this indicates an obstruction. This is a very serious condition and you must get medical help.

5. Laxity of the muscle between the stomach and the oesophagus may also result in vomiting but this time the milk will just ooze out. This type of vomiting can be controlled by giving small feeds, handling the baby carefully after feeds, and raising the upper part of his

body by placing a pillow *under* the mattress. This, too, is a condition that will improve in time.

6. *Illness.* Vomiting may be associated with an illness. It may occur after a bout of coughing, or when incubating an illness, or associated with diarrhoea, as in gastro-enteritis.

So, if your baby has any of the above symptoms, or seems to be ill, then consult your doctor.

There are many other less common causes of vomiting, so if in addition to vomiting the baby cries a lot and appears to be in pain or has a temperature, or even if he is just apathetic, then do consult your doctor.

What is mastitis?

Mastitis means inflammation of the breast.

It may be caused by an infection or by an injury. Even a kinked duct, and the resulting back-pressure, can cause it. It usually starts in one lobule but, if neglected, may spread to the whole breast, or develop into a localized breast abscess which may require a surgical incision.

If, on the other hand, it is treated immediately and intelligently, then the condition will subside within 1–2 days.

The first indication of the condition is a small red area on the breast which is tender to the touch.

What to do

1. Continue to breast-feed, but begin each feed on the affected side. Do not give any bottle-feeds.
2. While feeding lean forward and let the breast hang down so that gravity will help to drain it and to unkink the duct.
3. Apply frequent cold compresses to the tender area on the breast, as described on p. 31. Do this hourly or

2-hourly, if possible. This will give immediate relief.

4. Reduce your fluid intake temporarily, but do not deprive yourself of fluids altogether.

5. Do not wear any feeding bra which has flaps over cut-away centre portions because the edges of the cut-away part can compress ducts, cause back-pressure, and lead to inflammation.

6. If after a day the condition has not worsened, then it is resolving, and you should continue the above treatment for another day or two until it is back to normal.

7. If after a day's treatment the condition has worsened, then see your doctor who will prescribe an antibiotic. Continue with the above treatment in addition to taking the antibiotic and you will avert an abscess.

Can I continue to breast-feed if I get sick?

This to a large extent, depends on the type of illness, your physical condition, and how you feel. If you merely feel indisposed or have some minor illness you may continue to breast-feed. If, however, you develop a serious illness then your doctor will probably advise you to wean the baby.

Should you require minor surgery than you may arrange for the baby to be admitted with you to hospital and you can continue to breast-feed him. It may be necessary for the baby to be given one or two odd bottle-feeds until you recover from the anaesthetic.

In the case of a sudden emergency, requiring hospitalization and major surgery, the baby will have to be weaned.

It may interest you to know of one mother who developed polio when her baby was 6 months old. The baby refused to feed from a bottle or a cup and was very unhappy. This distressed the mother, so she was allowed to continue breast-feeding him. She was nursed at home, and the grandmother held the baby to the breast for feeds, as the mother could not lift her arms.

The baby did not contract polio, even though he was so young and was in such close contact with his mother during the incubation period and while she was ill. The mother recovered completely and continued to breast-feed until the baby was 8–9 months old.

The doctor, in permitting the mother to breast-feed, reasoned that as the baby had been in close contact with the mother during the incubation period and had not caught the disease it was safer for him to continue to receive protection through the breast-milk.

Another mother developed gastric flu when her baby was 4 weeks old. For 4 days she could neither eat nor drink, she had diarrhoea, and her temperature was just below 39·5° C. (104° F.). And yet she breast-fed her baby without any trouble. The baby flourished and did not catch the infection.

In the case of mental depression each case must be assessed individually. The general trend is to wean the baby quickly. But this may not be wise in the case of a woman who desperately wants to breast-feed. In such a case weaning may aggravate her condition and make her feel that she has failed her baby, or she may become more anxious because she was not considered well enough to breast-feed. Whereas, if she is allowed to breast-feed under supervision it would give her the incentive to get better and the reassurance that she is not too ill. Doing something positive for the baby would also help to restore her confidence and to aid her recovery.

Will any medicines that I take pass into the breast-milk?
No doubt some medicines do pass into the breast-milk but they are unlikely to harm the baby. Medicines are usually taken only for a short time, so effects, if any, will be transitory.

Be confident that the advantages of breast-feeding far outweigh any possible ill-effects, and anyway you cannot be absolutely sure that cow's milk—which is the alternative substance for feeding the baby—is entirely free of D.D.T. or other medications. (For example, cows are also given antibiotics when they have mastitis.)

What you can do
1. Take medicines only when necessary. Too many people tend to take medicines (e.g., aspirin, sleeping tablets, etc.) when not absolutely necessary.
2. Do not exceed the dose prescribed by the doctor.
3. Do not continue to take medicines for longer than recommended.

Note: I know one woman who conceived while she was being treated with cortisone for some chronic condition. She desperately wanted to breast-feed and was allowed to do so, even though she was still taking cortisone. She breast-fed successfully for 9 months. Her child, $2\frac{1}{2}$ years old at the time of writing, is quite well and, the mother maintains, much healthier than an older child who was not breast-fed. This she attributes to breast-feeding.

Is it true that a woman cannot conceive while she is breast-feeding?
In theory the pituitary hormones are supposed to suppress ovulation during lactation and sometimes they

do—this is why some women do not menstruate at all while they breast-feed.

But there are many women who do menstruate either regularly or infrequently, while completely breast-feeding a baby.

Obviously if a woman menstruates, then she also ovulates and she is therefore physically capable of conceiving. But even the woman who is not menstruating is capable of conceiving because she may ovulate spontaneously either when she has an orgasm or has intercourse, and this can even occur during the puerperium (the 6–8 weeks following the birth of the baby). Young women under 35 years of age are more prone to spontaneous ovulation than older women.

So do not rely on breast-feeding as a method of contraception.

Must I stop breast-feeding if I become pregnant again?
Women who are breast-feeding vary considerably as to when they begin to menstruate after the baby is born. Some begin almost immediately after the postnatal check-up (6–8 weeks after birth), and others do not menstruate at all while they are breast-feeding. Many will begin to menstruate somewhere between these two extremes. Some have odd periods and do not establish a proper cycle until after weaning.

Now, because one judges the onset of a pregnancy by the cessation of menstruation, it may take several months before you will definitely know that you are pregnant again.

Carry on breast-feeding until the pregnancy has been confirmed. Then it will depend on your physical condition whether you begin weaning immediately, or whether you continue to breast-feed for another few weeks, and so start weaning when your baby is 8 months old. What is very important is that you wean slowly (*see* p. 65).

(*see* p. 65)

QUOTE FROM A LETTER

'. . . She is just over the 9-month mark now . . . and I have just finished weaning her a week or so ago—on to a cup, of course, not a bottle. . . . Actually, one of the reasons why I got on with weaning her fairly promptly was that I discovered I was expecting another baby in October. I reckoned three months of keeping them both going was about enough!'

Can I breast-feed while I'm on the Pill?

The Pill is far from being the healthiest method of contraception, but you can still breast-feed if you are taking a low-oestrogen pill. A high oestrogen level in your body may inhibit prolactin before lactation is well established and therefore make breast-feeding more difficult, but it is unlikely to affect the milk-supply later, when the baby's sucking is strong enough to counteract its effect.

INDEX

INDEX

The Other Know-how Books

The Know-how of Infant Care
. . . should be bedside reading for all new mothers . . .
There are excellent sections on 'Should a child be obedient ?'
and 'How necessary is discipline ?' which, if learnt by
heart by every new mother, would go a long way towards
reducing the length of waiting lists for the child guidance
clinics . . . The last chapter consists of eleven 'Final do's
and don'ts' which are so useful and sensible that they
should be printed on large posters, and displayed
prominently in all baby clinics and paediatric departments.

Update

The Know-how of Infant Feeding
. . . the general approach to the baby and its feeding is
sensible, flexible and gay . . . It is an excellent book to offer
the young mother as it will induce the right unworrying
frame of mind and prevent unnecessary anxiety. It is
commended to health visitors, especially those who
recommend good ways and stick to them regardless of
fashion, as it will endorse their advice.

Nursing Mirror

The Know-how of Pregnancy and Labour
. . . questions are answered clearly in a commonsense man-
ner and the advice and explanations given are to the point,
dealing with the relevant needs of the expectant mother.

Health Visitor